91 Meal and Juice Recipes to Control Your Hunger after Having Quit Smoking:

Smart and Filling Foods That Will Compliment a Healthy Diet

By

Joe Correa CSN

COPYRIGHT

© 2017 Live Stronger Faster Inc.

This publication is designed to provide accurate and authoritative information in regard to the subject matter covered. It is sold with the understanding that neither the author nor the publisher is engaged in rendering medical advice. If medical advice or assistance is needed, consult with a doctor. This book is considered a guide and should not be used in any way detrimental to your health. Consult with a physician before starting this nutritional plan to make sure it's right for you.

ACKNOWLEDGEMENTS

This book is dedicated to my friends and family that have had mild or serious illnesses so that you may find a solution and make the necessary changes in your life.

91 Meal and Juice Recipes to Control Your Hunger after Having Quit Smoking:

Smart and Filling Foods That Will Compliment a Healthy Diet

By

Joe Correa CSN

CONTENTS

ABOUT THE AUTHOR

After years of Research, I honestly believe in the positive effects that proper nutrition can have over the body and mind. My knowledge and experience has helped me live healthier throughout the years and which I have shared with family and friends. The more you know about eating and drinking healthier, the sooner you will want to change your life and eating habits.

Nutrition is a key part in the process of being healthy and living longer so get started today. The first step is the most important and the most significant.

INTRODUCTION

91 Meal and Juice Recipes to Control Your Hunger after Having Quit Smoking: Smart and Filling Foods That Will Compliment a Healthy Diet

By Joe Correa CSN

An important issue related to this problem is a myth we've often heard: "If I quit smoking, I will probably start gaining weight! The problem is that all smokers are used to having something in their hands and mouth, and when they quit smoking, they turn to unhealthy snacks to keep their hands and mouth busy. This habit, naturally, leads to gaining weight, which is again related to smoking.

Food cravings are at a peak in the first few weeks of recovery. This is a crucial time to trick your organism and eliminate those feelings. It's no secret that smoking is one of the leading causes of death in the world. This habit has some devastating effects on the entire body, your immune system, respiratory tract, and even your cardiovascular system. Not to mention the effects cigarettes have on your skin, teeth, and nails. Unfortunately, we are all aware of these facts but somehow we still decide to start smoking hoping that it won't happen to us.

This book offers you exactly that! Plenty of healthy recipes that will definitely control your food cravings and keep your organism balanced. The recipes inside like: "Barley Porridge" or "Green Apple Overnight Oats with Raisins" are full of precious fibers and the perfect way to start your new, healthy, and smoke-free day. Start today and be consistent to see the results you truly want.

91 MEAL AND JUICE RECIPES TO CONTROL YOUR HUNGER AFTER HAVING QUIT SMOKING: SMART AND FILLING FOODS THAT WILL COMPLIMENT A HEALTHY DIET

JUICES

1.   Cranberry Pineapple Juice

Ingredients:

1 cup of cranberries

1 cup of pineapple, chopped

1 medium-sized apple, chopped

1 cup of apricot, sliced

Preparation:

Using a large colander, rinse the cranberries under cold running water. Drain and fill the measuring cup. Reserve the rest for later.

Using a sharp cutting knife, cut the top and peel the

pineapple. Chop into small cubes and fill the measuring cup. Reserve the rest in the refrigerator for some other juice.

Wash the apple and cut in half. Remove the core and cut into bite-sized pieces. Set aside.

Wash the apricot and cut in half. Remove the pit and chop into small pieces. Set aside.

Now, combine cranberries, pineapple, apple, and apricot in a juicer. Process until well juiced. Transfer to a serving glass and add some ice cubes.

Serve immediately.

Nutrition information per serving: Kcal: 248, Protein: 4.3g, Carbs: 76.1g, Fats: 1.3g

2.   Cauliflower Broccoli Juice

Ingredients:

1 cup of cauliflower, chopped

2 cups of broccoli, chopped

1 cup of asparagus, trimmed and chopped

2 oz of coconut water

Preparation:

Trim off the outer leaves of the cauliflower. Chop into small pieces and fill the measuring cup. Reserve the rest for later.

Wash the broccoli and trim off the outer leaves. Chop into small pieces and fill the measuring cup. Reserve the rest in the refrigerator.

Wash the asparagus and trim off the woody ends. Chop into small pieces and fill the measuring cup. Set aside.

Now, combine cauliflower, broccoli, and asparagus in a juicer. Process until well juiced. Transfer to a serving glass and stir in the coconut water.

Refrigerate for 10-15 minutes before serving.

Enjoy!

Nutrition information per serving: Kcal: 390, Protein: 8.7g, Carbs: 43.9g, Fats: 34.5g

3.   Cinnamon Banana Juice

Ingredients:

1 large banana, peeled and chunked

1 medium-sized Red Delicious apple, cored

1 whole plum, cored

¼ tsp of cinnamon, ground

2 oz of coconut water

Preparation:

Peel the banana and cut into small chunks. Set aside. Wash the apple and cut lengthwise in half. Remove the core and cut into bite-sized pieces. Set aside.

Wash the plum and cut in half. Remove the pit and cut into bite-sized pieces. Set aside.

Now, combine banana, apple, and plum in a juicer and process until well juiced. Transfer to a serving glass and stir in the coconut water and cinnamon.

Add few ice cubes before serving and enjoy!

Nutrition information per serving: Kcal: 238, Protein: 2.5g, Carbs: 68.4g, Fats: 1.1g

4. Cucumber Honey Juice

Ingredients:

1 medium-sized cucumber, sliced

1 tbsp honey, raw

1 cup of strawberries, chopped

1 cup of spinach, torn

2 oz of water

Preparation:

Wash the cucumber and cut into thin slices.

Wash the strawberries and remove the stems. Cut into bite-sized pieces and set aside.

Wash the spinach thoroughly under cold running water. Slightly drain and torn into small pieces. Set aside.

Now, combine cucumber, strawberries, and spinach in a juicer and process until juiced. Transfer to a serving glass and stir in the water and honey.

Garnish with some mint, but it's optional.

Refrigerate for 10 minutes before serving.

Enjoy!

Nutrition information per serving: Kcal: 83, Protein: 6.9g, Carbs: 24.6g, Fats: 1.3g

5.   Apricot Cucumber Juice

Ingredients:

1 cup of apricots

1 large cucumber, sliced

1 cup of pineapple, chunked

1 cup of fresh spinach, torn

1 whole lemon

½ cup of raw broccoli, chopped

½ cup of pure coconut water

Preparation:

Wash the apricots and cut in half. Remove the pit and chop into chunks. Set aside.

Wash the cucumber and chop into thick slices. Set aside.

Cut the top of a pineapple and peel it using a sharp knife. Cut into small chunks and reserve the rest in the refrigerator.

Peel the lemon and cut lengthwise in half. Set aside.

Combine spinach and broccoli in a colander and wash

under cold running water. Drain and roughly chop. Set aside.

Now, process apricots, cucumber, pineapple, lemon, spinach, and broccoli in a juicer. Transfer to serving glasses and stir in the coconut water.

Add some ice and serve immediately.

Nutrition information per serving: Kcal: 218, Protein: 10g, Carbs: 64g, Fats: 1.9g

6.   Asparagus Collard Greens Juice

Ingredients:

1 cup of fresh asparagus, chopped

1 cup of collard greens, torn

1 large peach, chopped

1 large grapefruit, peeled

1 cup of Romaine lettuce, shredded

1 cup of fennel, sliced

Preparation:

Wash the asparagus and trim off the woody ends. Chop into small pieces and set aside.

Combine collard greens and lettuce in a colander and wash under cold running water. Torn with hands and set aside.

Wash the peach and cut in half. Remove the pit and cut into bite-sized pieces. Set aside.

Peel the grapefruit and cut into small pieces. Set aside.

Wash the fennel bulb and trim off the wilted outer layers. Cut into small chunks and set aside.

Now, combine asparagus, collard greens, peach, lettuce, grapefruit, and fennel in a juicer and process until juiced.

Transfer to serving glasses and add some ice before serving.

Nutrition information per serving: Kcal: 187, Protein: 9.1g, Carbs: 57.9g, Fats: 1.4g

7.   Blackberry Turnip Juice

Ingredients:

1 cup of fresh blackberries

1 cup of turnip greens, chopped

1 cup of plums, halved

½ tsp of ginger, ginger

1 tsp of coconut sugar

½ cup of water

Preparation:

Wash the blackberries under cold running water. Set aside.

Wash the turnip greens and torn with hands. Set aside.

Wash the plums and cut in half. Remove the pits and set aside.

Now, combine blackberries, turnip greens, and plums in a juicer. Process until juiced.

Transfer to a serving glass and stir in the coconut sugar, ginger, and water.

Refrigerate for 10 minutes before serving.

Enjoy!

Nutrition information per serving: Kcal: 141, Protein: 4.2g, Carbs: 40.3g, Fats: 1.4g

8.   Orange Radish Juice

Ingredients:

1 large orange, peeled

1 cup of radishes, chopped

1 medium-sized apple, peeled and wedged

1 cup of Iceberg lettuce, torn

1 cup of watercress, chopped

1 tbsp of honey, raw

Preparation:

Peel the orange and divide into wedges. Set aside.

Wash the radishes and trim off the green parts. Cut into small pieces and fill the measuring cup. Set aside.

Wash the apple and cut in half. Remove the core and chop into small pieces. Set aside.

Rinse the lettuce and watercress. Drain and torn with hands.

Now, combine orange, radishes, apple, lettuce, and watercress in a juicer and process until juiced.

Transfer to serving glasses and add some ice before serving.

Enjoy!

Nutrition information per serving: Kcal: 150, Protein: 7.3g, Carbs: 53.4g, Fats: 0.8g

9.   Cranberry Honey Juice

Ingredients:

1 cup of fresh cranberries

1 tbsp of honey, raw

2 cups of cherries, pitted

1 cup of leek, chopped

1 tbsp of fresh mint, finely chopped

Preparation:

Rinse the cranberries and cherries under cold running water using a colander. Drain and set aside.

Cut the cheries into halves. Remove the pits and set aside.

Wash the leek and cut into small pieces. Set aside.

Combine cranberries, cherries, leek, and mint in a juicer and process until juiced.

Transfer to serving glasses and stir in the honey.

Add some ice and serve!

Nutrition information per serving: Kcal: 248, Protein: 5g, Carbs: 75.5g, Fats: 1g

10.   Coco Apricot Juice

Ingredients:

1 cup of apricots, sliced

½ cup of pure coconut water, unsweetened

1 tbsp of coconut sugar

1 cup of mango, chopped

Preparation:

Wash the apricots and cut in half. Remove the pits and chop into small pieces. Set aside.

Peel the mango and cut into small chunks. Fill the measuring cup and rserve the rest in the refrigerator.

Now, combine apricots, mango, and coconut water in a juicer. Process until juiced.

Transfer to serving glasses and stir in the coconut sugar.

Add few ice cubes and serve immediately.

Nutrition information per serving: Kcal: 155, Protein: 3.6g, Carbs: 43g, Fats: 1.2g

11.　Cauliflower Fennel Juice

Ingredients:

1 cup of cauliflower, chopped

1 cup of fennel, sliced

1 cup of beet greens, chopped

1 cup of celery, chopped

1 cup of red leaf lettuce, shredded

1 cup of romaine lettuce, shredded

1 large grapefruit

½ cup of pure coconut water

1 tsp of honey

Preparation:

Trim off the outer leaves of cauliflower. Wash it and cut into small pieces. Reserve the rest in the refrigerator.

Wash the fennel bulb and trim off the wilted outer layers. Cut into small chunks and set aside.

Combine beet greens, red leaf lettuce, and Romaine lettuce in a colander and wash under cold running water.

Drain and chop roughly with hands. Set aside.

Peel the grapefruit and divide into wedges. Set aside.

Wash the celery and cut into small pieces. set aside.

Now, process cauliflower, fennel, beet greens, celery, lettuce, and grapefruit in a juicer. Transfer to serving glasses and stir in the coconut water and honey.

Add some ice and serve!

Nutrition information per serving: Kcal: 163, Protein: 8.3g, Carbs: 56.3g, Fats: 1.2g

12. Spinach Peach Juice

Ingredients:

1 large peach, chopped

1 cup of baby spinach, torn

2 large Golden delicious apples, peeled and seeds removed

½ cup of water

1 large carrot, sliced

½ whole lemon

Preparation:

Wash the peach and cut in half. Remove the pit and chop into small pieces. Set aside.

Wash the baby spinach thoroughly and torn with hands. Set aside.

Wash the apples and cut in half. Remove the core and cut into bite-sized pieces. Set aside.

Wash the carrot and cut into thick slices. Set aside.

Peel the lemon and cut lengthwise in half. Reserve the rest for later.

Now, combine peach, spinach, apples, peach, carrot, and lemon in a juicer and process until juiced.

Transfer to serving glasses and refrigerate for 10 minutes before serving.

Nutrition information per serving: Kcal: 297, Protein: 5.5g, Carbs: 87.5g, Fats: 1.5g

13.   Banana Spinach Juice

Ingredients:

1 large banana, peeled

1 cup of spinach, torn

2 whole lemons, peeled

1 slice of ginger root, peeled

1 tsp of honey

Preparation:

Peel the banana and chop into chunks. Set aside.

Rinse the spinach thoroughly under cold running water using a colander. Drain and torn with hands. Set aside.

Peel the lemons and cut lengthwise in half. Set aside.

Peel the ginger root and finely chop it. Set aside.

Combine banana, spinach, lemons, and ginger in a juicer and process until juiced.

Transfer to serving glasses and stir in the honey.

Add some ice and serve.

Nutrition information per serving: Kcal: 139, Protein: 4.5g, Carbs: 44.4g, Fats: 1.2g

14.   Kiwi Apple Juice

Ingredients:

2 large kiwis, peeled

1 medium-sized apple, cored

1 cup of fresh spinach

1 large cucumber

1 small ginger root slice, 1-inch

Preparation:

Peel the kiwis and cut lengthwise in half. Set aside.

Wash the apple and remove the core. Cut into bite-sized pieces and set aside.

Wash the spinach thoroughly and torn with hands. Set aside.

Wash the cucumber and cut into thick slices. Set aside.

Peel the ginger root slice and set aside.

Now, process spinach, kiwis, apple, cucumber and ginger in a juicer.

Transfer to a serving glass and add some ice before serving.

Nutrition information per serving: Kcal: 201, Protein: 13.2g, Carbs: 56.5g, Fats: 2.6g

15.   Strawberry Orange Juice

Ingredients:

1 cup of fresh strawberries

1 large orange, peeled

1 cup of fresh cranberries

2 oz of coconut water

Preparation:

Combine strawberries and cranberries in a colander and wash under cold running water. Drain and set aside.

Peel the orange and divide into wedges. Set aside.

Combine cranberries, strawberries, and orange in a juicer and process until juiced.

Transfer to serving glasses and stir in the coconut water.

Add some ice and serve immediately.

Nutrition information per serving: Kcal: 137, Protein: 3.1g, Carbs: 46.7g, Fats: 0.7g

16.   Watermelon Honey Juice

Ingredients:

1 cup of watermelon, seeded

1 tbsp of liquid honey

1 cup of fresh blueberries

1 cup of fresh raspberries

1 cup of fresh cranberries

1 large lemon, peeled

Preparation:

Cut the watermelon lengthwise. For one cup, you will need about 1 large wedge. Peel and cut into chunks. Remove the seeds and set aside. Reserve the rest of the melon for some other juices.

Combine blueberries, raspberries, and cranberries in a colander and wash under cold running water. Drain and set aside.

Peel the lemon and cut lengthwise in half. Set aside.

Now, process watermelon, blueberries, raspberries, cranberries, and lemon in a juicer. Transfer to serving glasses and stir in the liquid honey.

Add some ice cubes before serving.

Enjoy!

Nutrition information per serving: Kcal: 230, Protein: 4.1g, Carbs: 53.1g, Fats: 1.7g

17.   Ginger Squash Juice

Ingredients:

1 tsp of ginger, ground

1 cup of acorn squash, cubed

1 cup of pumpkin, cubed

1 cup of butternut squash, cubed

1 large cucumber

Preparation:

Wash the crookneck squash and cut in half. Scoop out the seeds using a spoon. Cut into small chunks and set aside. Reserve the rest for another juice.

Peel the pumpkin and cut in half. Scoop out the seeds using a spoon. Cut one large wedge and peel it. Cut into small chunks and set aside. Reserve the rest for later.

Peel the butternut squash and remove the seeds using a spoon. Cut into small cubes and reserve the rest of the squash for some other recipe. Wrap in a plastic foil and refrigerate.

Wash the cucumber and cut into thick slices. Set aside.

Now, combine crookneck squash, pumpkin, butternut squash, and cucumber in a juicer and process until juiced. Transfer to serving glasses and stir in the ginger.

Add some ice and serve immediately.

Nutrition information per serving: Kcal: 140, Protein: 5.8g, Carbs: 40.1g, Fats: 0.9g

18.   Kale Watercress Juice

Ingredients:

1 fennel bulb, trimmed

1 cup of fresh kale

1 cup of watercress

1 cup of fresh basil

1 large cucumber

3 tbsp of fresh parsley

A handful of spinach

Preparation:

Combine kale, watercress, basil, parsley, and spinach in a colander and wash under cold running water. Drain and torn with hands. Set aside.

Wash the fennel bulb and trim off the wilted outer layers. Cut into small chunks and set aside.

Wash the cucumber and cut into thick slices. Set aside.

Now, process kale, watercress, fennel, basil, parsley, spinach, and cucumber in a juicer.

Transfer to serving glasses and stir in the Cayenne pepper. You can add some salt but this is optional.

Refrigerate for 10 minutes before serving.

Nutrition information per serving: Kcal: 280, Protein: 6.1g, Carbs: 84.2g, Fats: 1.3g

19.   Tomato Beet Juice

Ingredients:

1 medium-sized Roma tomato, chopped

1 cup of beets, trimmed

1 cup of fresh basil, torn

1 tsp of ginger, ground

1 tbsp of fresh parsley, chopped

Preparation:

Wash the tomato and place in a bowl. Cut into quarters and reserve the juice while cutting. Set aside.

Wash the beets and trim off the green parts. Cut into small pieces and set aside.

Wash the basil thoroughly and torn with hands. Set aside.

Now, process tomato, beets, basil, and ginger in a juicer.

Transfer to a serving glass and refrigerate for 10 minutes before serving.

Enjoy!

Nutrition information per serving: Kcal: 99, Protein: 6.4g, Carbs: 28.7g, Fats: 1.2g

20.   Cherry Apple Juice

Ingredients:

1 cup of fresh cherries, pitted

2 large red apples, cored

1 large banana, chopped

1 cup of watercress

A handful of fresh spinach

Preparation:

Wash the cherries under cold running water. Drain and cut in half. Remove the pits and set aside.

Wash the apple and cut in half. Remove the core and chop into small pieces. Set aside.

Peel the banana and cut into small chunks. Set aside.

Combine watercress and spinach in a colander and wash thoroughly. Torn with hands and set aside.

Now, combine cherries, apples, banana, watercress, and spinach in a juicer and process until juiced.

Transfer to serving glasses and add few ice cubes before serving.

Enjoy!

Nutrition information per serving: Kcal: 390, Protein: 6.6g, Carbs: 113g, Fats: 1.7g

21.　Zucchini Watermelon Juice

Ingredients:

1 medium-sized zucchini, peeled and chopped

1 cup of watermelon, diced

2 cups of green grapes

1 slice of ginger, 1-inch

1 tbsp of fresh mint, finely chopped

Preparation:

Wash the zucchini and cut in half. Scoop out the seeds using a spoon. Cut into small chunks and set aside.

Cut the watermelon lengthwise. For one cup, you will need about one large wedge. Peel and cut into chunks. Remove the seeds and set aside. Reserve the rest of the melon for some other juices.

Wash the grapes under cold running water. Drain and set aside.

Peel the ginger slice and set aside.

Now, process zucchini, watermelon, grapes, and ginger in a juicer.

Transfer to serving glasses and garnish with mint.

Refrigerate for 10 minutes before serving.

Nutrition information per serving: Kcal: 308, Protein: 5.7g, Carbs: 81.3g, Fats: 2.1g

22.   Apple Yam Juice

Ingredients:

2 medium-sized green apples, cored

1 small sweet potato, peeled

2 large carrots, sliced

1 large orange, peeled

¼ tsp of pumpkin pie spice

Preparation:

Wash the apples and cut in half. Remove the core and chop into bite-sized pieces. Set aside.

Peel the potato and place in a pot of boiling water. Cook for 5 minutes, or until soften. Remove from the heat and drain. Set aside to cool.

Wash the carrot and cut into thin slices. Set aside.

Peel the orange and divide into wedges. Cut each wedge in half and set aside.

Now, combine apples, potato, carrot, and orange in a juicer. Process until juiced. Transfer to serving glasses and stir in the pumpkin spice.

Add some ice cubes and serve immediately.

Enjoy!

Nutrition information per serving: Kcal: 147, Protein: 2.1g, Carbs: 35.4g, Fats: 0.1g

23.   Apple Chia Juice

Ingredients:

2 large apples, cored

1 tbsp of chia seeds

3 large carrots, sliced

½ tsp of ginger, ground

Preparation:

Wash the apples. Cut in half and remove the core. Cut into bite-sized pieces and set aside.

Wash and cut the carrots into thin slices. Set aside.

Now, process in a juicer until well juiced. Transfer to serving glasses and stir in the chia seeds.

Refrigerate for 10 minutes to allow chia to soak up the liquid. Add a little bit of water to adjust the thickness, if needed.

Enjoy!

Nutrition information per serving: Kcal: 177, Protein: 3.2g, Carbs: 28.4g, Fats: 4.6g

24.   Squash Broccoli Juice

Ingredients:

½ yellow squash, peeled and chopped

1 medium-sized broccoli, chopped

½ cup of fresh kale

1 large apple, cored

¼ cup of fresh spinach

4 small carrots

Preparation:

Peel the squash and cut in half. Scoop out the seeds and chop into bite-sized pieces. Reserve the remaining half in the refrigerator.

Wash and chop the broccoli and carrots. Combine it with squash.

Wash and core the apple. Chop into bite-sized pieces and add to the remaining prepared ingredients.

Combine spinach and kale in a medium bowl and add water enough to cover it. Soak for 15 minutes.

Now, combine squash, broccoli, apple, and carrots in a

juicer. Drain the kale and spinach and add it to the juicer. Process until well juiced.

Transfer to serving glasses and refrigerate for 10 minutes before serving.

Enjoy!

Nutrition information per serving: Kcal: 81, Protein: 2.3g, Carbs: 18.4g, Fats: 0.2g

25. Cucumber Celery Juice

Ingredients:

1 large cucumber, sliced

1 celery stalk, chopped

½ cup of fresh kale

1 large lime, peeled

Preparation:

Wash and chop the cucumber and celery. Add it to the bowl with lime.

Soak the kale in water for 15 minutes. Set aside.

Peel the lime and cut into bite-sized pieces. Place it in a bowl and set aside.

Drain the kale and process it with cucumber, lime, and celery.

Transfer to serving glasses and refrigerate for a while, or add some ice and serve immediately.

Nutrition information per serving: Kcal: 171, Protein: 3.2g, Carbs: 47.3g, Fats: 1.3g

26.   Pear Lime Juice

Ingredients:

1 large pear, cored

1 lime, peeled

1 cup of green grapes

2 large cucumbers, sliced

Preparation:

Wash the pear and remove the core. Cut into bite-sized pieces and set aside.

Peel the lime and cut into quarters. Set aside.

Wash the green grapes under cold running water and drain using colander. Set aside.

Wash the cucumbers and cut into thin slices. Set aside.

Now, combine pear, lime, grapes and cucumber in a juicer. Process until juiced. Transfer to serving glasses and stir well.

Refrigerate for 10 minutes before serving.

Enjoy!

Nutrition information per serving: Kcal: 113, Protein: 18.3g, Carbs: 31.3g, Fats: 0.1g

27.   Carrot Lemon Juice

Ingredients:

3 large carrots, sliced

1 large lemon, peeled

1 medium-sized cucumber, sliced

1 large pear, cored

¼ cup of fresh mint

½ cup of broccoli, chopped

1 small ginger root slice, 1-inch

½ tsp of green tea powder

2 oz of water

Preparation:

Wash the carrots and cut into small pieces. Set aside.

Peel the lemon and cut into quarters. Set aside.

Wash and cut the cucumber into small pieces. Set aside.

Wash the pear and remove the core. Cut into bite-sized pieces and set aside.

Combine broccoli and mint in a colander and wash under cold running water. Drain and set aside.

Peel the ginger root and set aside.

Combine tea powder and hot water in a small cup. Let it stand for 5 minutes.

Now, combine carrots, lemon, cucumber, pear, mint, broccoli, and ginger root slice in a juicer. Process until nicely juiced.

Transfer to serving glasses and stir in the tea mixture.

Refrigerate for 5 minutes before serving.

Nutrition information per serving: Kcal: 141, Protein: 5.5g, Carbs: 45.7g, Fats: 0.9g

28.   Strawberry Carrot Juice

Ingredients:

1 cup of fresh strawberries, chopped

1 large carrot, sliced

1 medium-sized green apple, cored and chopped

1 medium orange, wedged

1 cup of cucumber, sliced

Preparation:

Wash the strawberries and remove the top stems. Cut into small pieces and set aside.

Wash the carrot and cut into thin slices. Set aside.

Wash the apple and cut in half. Remove the core and cut into bite-sized pieces. Set aside.

Peel the orange and divide into wedges. Set aside.

Wash the cucumber and cut into thin slices. Set aside.

Now, process strawberries, carrots, apple, orange, and cucumber in a juicer. Transfer to the serving glasses refrigerate for 5 minutes before serving.

Enjoy!

Nutrition information per serving: Kcal: 104, Protein: 3.9g, Carbs: 31.2g, Fats: 1.1g

29. Cucumber Apple Juice

Ingredients:

1 large cucumber, sliced

1 large red apple, cored

2 medium-sized beets, trimmed

1 large lime, peeled

¼ tsp of ginger, ground

Preparation:

Wash the cucumber and cut it into thick slices. Set aside.

Wash the apple and remove the core. Cut into bite-sized pieces and set aside.

Wash the beets and trim off the green ends. Save it for another juice. Cut the beet into small pieces. Set aside.

Peel the lime and cut into quarters. Set aside.

Now, process cucumber, apple, beets, and lime in a juicer. Transfer to serving glasses and add some ice before serving.

Enjoy!

Nutrition information per serving: Kcal: 109, Protein: 2.8g, Carbs: 33.6g, Fats: 0.7g

30.   Apple Lemon Juice

Ingredients:

1 green apple, cored

1 large lemon, peeled

1 large broccoli, chopped

1 large cucumber, sliced

¼ tsp of peppermint extract

½ cup of fresh mint

Preparation:

Wash the apple and remove the core. Cut into bite-sized pieces and set aside.

Peel the lemon and cut into quarters. Set aside.

Wash the broccoli and cut into small pieces. Set aside.

Wash the cucumber and cut into thick slices. Set aside.

Wash the fresh mint and soak in water for 5 minutes.

Now, combine apple, lemon, broccoli, cucumber, and mint in a juicer and process until juiced.

Transfer to serving glasses and stir in the peppermint

extract.

Garnish with some extra mint leaves and add some ice before serving.

Enjoy!

Nutrition information per serving: Kcal: 191, Protein: 2.3g, Carbs: 28.4g, Fats: 1.7g

31.   Apricot Pomegranate Juice

Ingredients:

2 large apricots, pitted

1 cup of pomegranate seeds

2 large oranges, peeled

1 cup of green grapes

1 large lemon, peeled

1 small ginger slice, peeled

Preparation:

Wash the apricots and cut in half. Remove the pits and cut into small pieces. Set aside.

Cut the top of the pomegranate fruit using a sharp knife. Slice down to each of the white membranes inside of the fruit. Pop the seeds into a measuring cup and set aside.

Peel the oranges and divide into wedges. Set aside.

Peel the lemon and cut lengthwise in half. Set aside.

Peel the ginger slice and set aside.

Now, combine apricots, pomegranate, oranges, lemon, and

ginger in a juicer. Process until well juiced and transfer to serving glasses. Refrigerate for 20 minutes before serving.

Nutrition information per serving: Kcal: 294, Protein: 7.2g, Carbs: 88.9g, Fats: 2.3g

32.   Apple Cucumber Juice

Ingredients:

1 large red apple, cored

1 large cucumber, sliced

1 cup of blueberries

1 cup of fresh mint, torn

2 oz of coconut water

Preparation:

Wash the apple and cut in half. Remove the core and cut into bite-sized pieces. Set aside.

Wash the cucumber and gently peel it. Cut into thin slices and set aside.

Place the blueberries in a colander and wash under cold running water. Drain and set aside.

Wash the mint thoroughly and torn with hands. Set aside.

Now, combine apple, cucumber, blueberries, and mint in a juicer. Process until juiced and transfer to serving glasses. Stir in the coconut water and refrigerate for 10 minutes, or add some ice before serving.

Enjoy!

Nutrition information per serving: Kcal: 258, Protein: 4.7g, Carbs: 74.6g, Fats: 1.6g

33.   Raspberry Kiwi Juice

Ingredients:

1 cup of raspberries

1 large kiwi, peeled

2 cups of watermelon, chopped

1 large orange, peeled

2 oz coconut water

Preparation:

Wash the raspberries thoroughly under cold running water. Drain and set aside.

Peel the kiwi and cut lengthwise in half. Set aside.

Cut the watermelon lengthwise. For two cups, you will need about two large wedges. Peel and cut into chunks. Remove the seeds and set aside. Reserve the rest of the melon for some other juices. Set aside.

Peel the orange and divide into wedges. Set aside.

Now, combine raspberries, kiwi, watermelon, and orange in a juicer. Process until juiced and transfer to serving glasses. Stir in the coconut water and refrigerate for 10

minutes before serving.

Nutrition information per serving: Kcal: 232, Protein: 5.8g, Carbs: 71.4g, Fats: 1.8g

34.   Parsnip Parsley Juice

Ingredients:

1 cup of parsnip, sliced

1 tbsp of fresh parsley, chopped

3 large red bell peppers, chopped

1 cup of butternut squash, cubed

2 oz of water

Preparation:

Wash the parsnip and peel it. Cut into thin slices and set aside.

Wash the red bell peppers and cut lengthwise in half. Remove the seeds and chop into small pieces.

Peel the butternut squash and remove the seeds using a spoon. Cut into small cubes and fill the measuring cup. Reserve the rest of the squash for some other recipe. Wrap in a plastic foil and refrigerate.

Now, combine parsnip, parsley, bell peppers, and butternut squash in a juicer. Process until well juiced and transfer to serving glasses. Stir in the water and add some ice.

Serve immediately.

Nutrition information per serving: Kcal: 238, Protein: 7.9g, Carbs: 70.2g, Fats: 2.1g

35.   Pomegranate Apple Juice

Ingredients:

1 cup of pomegranate seeds

1 large green apple, cored and chopped

1 large papaya, peeled and chopped

1 tbsp of fresh mint, chopped

2 oz of water

Preparation:

Cut the top of the pomegranate fruit using a sharp knife. Slice down to each of the white membranes inside of the fruit. Pop the seeds into a measuring cup and set aside.

Wash the apple and cut in half. Using a sharp knife, remove the core and cut into bite-sized pieces. Set aside.

Peel the papaya and cut lengthwise in half. Scoop out the black seeds and flesh using a spoon. Cut into small chunks and set aside.

Now, combine pomegranate, apple, papaya, and mint in a juicer. Process until well juiced and transfer to serving glasses. Stir in the water and refrigerate for 10 minutes before serving.

Enjoy!

Nutrition information per serving: Kcal: 438, Protein: 6.1g, Carbs: 129g, Fats: 3.4g

36.   Lime Guava Juice

Ingredients:

1 cup of pineapple chunks

2 large limes, peeled

1 cup of guava, chopped

1 large cucumber, sliced

1 tbsp of fresh basil, chopped

2 oz of water

Preparation:

Peel the limes and cut lengthwise in half. Set aside.

Wash the guava and cut into chunks. Fill the measuring cup and reserve the rest for some other recipe in a refrigerator.

Cut the top of a pineapple and peel it using a sharp knife. Cut into small chunks and fill the measuring cup. Reserve the rest of the pineapple in a refrigerator.

Wash the cucumber and cut into thin slices. Set aside.

Now, combine limes, guava, pineapple, cucumber, and basil in a juicer. Process until well juiced and transfer to serving glasses. Stir in the water and refrigerate for 10

minutes before serving.

Nutrition information per serving: Kcal: 158, Protein: 4.7g, Carbs: 47.9g, Fats: 1.1g

37.   Apple Nutmeg Juice

Ingredients:

1 large green apple, cored

¼ tsp of nutmeg, ground

1 cup of cranberries

1 large pear, cored

3 large strawberries, chopped

1 large orange, peeled

2 oz of coconut water

Preparation:

Wash the apple and cut in half. Remove the core and cut into bite-sized pieces. Set aside.

Wash the cranberries thoroughly under cold running water. Drain and set aside.

Wash the pear and cut lengthwise in half. Remove the core and cut into bite-sized pieces. Set aside.

Wash the strawberries thoroughly and chop into small pieces. Set aside.

Peel the orange and divide into wedges. Set aside.

Now, combine pear, apple, strawberries, orange, and nutmeg in a juicer. Process until well juiced and transfer to serving glasses.

Stir in the water and refrigerate or add some ice before serving.

Nutrition information per serving: Kcal: 158, Protein: 4.7g, Carbs: 47.9g, Fats: 1.1g

38.   Collard Greens Watercress Juice

Ingredients:

1 cup of collard greens, torn

1 cup of watercress, torn

1 cup of asparagus, trimmed

1 green bell pepper, chopped

1 large cucumber, sliced

2 oz of water

¼ tsp of salt

Preparation:

Combine collard greens and watercress in a colander. Wash thoroughly under cold running water and torn with hands. Set aside.

Wash the asparagus and trim off the woody ends. Cut into bite-sized pieces and fill the measuring cup. Reserve the rest for some other juice.

Wash the bell pepper and lengthwise in half. Remove the seeds and chop into small pieces. Set aside.

Wash the cucumber and cut into thin slices. Set aside.

Now, combine collard greens, watercress, asparagus, bell pepper, and cucumber in a juicer and process until well juiced. Transfer to serving glasses and stir in the salt and water.

Refrigerate for 10 minutes before serving.

Nutrition information per serving: Kcal: 86, Protein: 8.2g, Carbs: 26.1g, Fats: 1g

39.   Swiss Chard Lettuce Juice

Ingredients:

1 cup of Swiss chard, torn

1 cup of red leaf lettuce, torn

1 cup of sweet potatoes, peeled

1 large fennel, chopped

1 cup of fresh spinach, torn

1 small cauliflower head, chopped

1 large lemon, peeled

Preparation:

Combine Swiss chard, red leaf lettuce, and spinach in a colander. Wash under cold running water and drain. Torn with hands and set aside.

Peel the sweet potato and cut into small chunks. Fill the measuring cup and reserve the rest for some other juice.

Wash the fennel bulb and trim off the wilted outer layers. Cut into small chunks and set aside.

Trim off the outer leaves of cauliflower. Wash it and cut into small pieces. Set aside.

Peel the lemon and cut lengthwise in half. Set aside.

Now, combine Swiss chard, lettuce, potato, fennel, cauliflower, and lemon in a juicer and process until well juiced. Transfer to serving glasses and add some ice before serving.

Nutrition information per serving: Kcal: 218, Protein: 14.3g, Carbs: 67.7g, Fats: 1.9g

40.   Pepper Cucumber Juice

Ingredients:

1 large yellow bell pepper, chopped

1 large cucumber, sliced

1 medium-sized fennel bulb, chopped

1 cup of Brussels sprouts, halved

¼ tsp of salt

2 oz of water

Preparation:

Wash the bell pepper and cut lengthwise in half. Remove the seeds and chop into small pieces. Set aside.

Wash the cucumber and cut into thin slices. Set aside.

Trimm off the fennel stalks and wilted outer layers. Cut into bite-sized pieces and set aside.

Trim off the outer leaves and wash the Brussels sprouts. Cut in half and set aside.

Now, combine bell peppers, cucumber, fennel, and Brussels sprouts in a juicer. Process until well juiced and stir in the salt and water. Refrigerate for 5 minutes before serving.

Nutrition information per serving: Kcal: 151, Protein: 9.7g, Carbs: 47.6g, Fats: 1.4g

41.   Blackberry Cucumber Juice

Ingredients:

1 cup of blackberries

1 large cucumber, sliced

5 whole plums, pitted

1 cup of purple cabbage, chopped

2 oz of water

Preparation:

Wash the blackberries under cold running water using a colander. Slightly drain and set aside.

Wash the cucumber and cut into thin slices. Set aside.

Wash the plums and cut in half. Remove the pits and cut into quarters. Set aside.

Wash the cabbage thoroughly under cold running water. Drain and roughly chop it. Set aside.

Now, combine plums, cabbage, blackberries, and cucumber in a juicer and process until juice. Transfer to serving glasses and stir in the water.

Refrigerate for 10 minutes before serving.

Nutrition information per serving: Kcal: 221, Protein: 7.5g, Carbs: 69.1g, Fats: 2.1g

42.   Beet Basil Juice

Ingredients:

1 cup of beets, chopped

1 cup of fresh basil, torn

2 cups of raspberries

1 large green apple, cored

1 large lemon, peeled

3 oz of water

Preparation:

Wash the beets and trim off the green ends. Cut into small pieces and fill the measuring cup. Reserve the greens for some other juice.

Wash the basil thoroughly under cold running water and torn with hands. Set aside.

Wash the raspberries under cold running water using a colander. Drain and set aside.

Wash the apple and cut in half. Remove the core and cut into bite-sized pieces. Set aside.

Peel the lemon and cut lengthwise in half. Set aside.

Now, combine beets, basil, raspberries, apple, and lemon in a juicer. Process until well juiced.

Stir in the water and refrigerate for 5 minutes before serving.

Enjoy!

Nutrition information per serving: Kcal: 218, Protein: 7.5g, Carbs: 76.4g, Fats: 2.5g

43.   Pomegranate Lemon Juice

Ingredients:

1 cup of pomegranate seeds

1 large lemon, peeled

1 large apricot, pitted

1 large orange, wedged

1 large carrot, peeled

2 oz of coconut water

Preparation:

Cut the top of the pomegranate fruit using a sharp knife. Slice down to each of the white membranes inside of the fruit. Pop the seeds into measuring cup and set aside.

Peel the lemon and cut lengthwise in half. Set aside.

Wash the apricot and cut in half. Remove the pit and cut into small pieces. Set aside.

Peel the orange and divide into wedges. Set aside.

Peel and wash the carrot. Cut into thin slices and set aside.

Now, combine pomegranate seeds, lemon, apricot, orange,

and carrot in a juicer. Process until well juiced and transfer to serving glasses. Stir in the coconut water and add few ice cubes before serving.

Nutrition information per serving: Kcal: 241, Protein: 7.3g, Carbs: 73.9g, Fats: 2.3g

44.   Kale Parsley Juice

Ingredients:

1 cup of fresh kale, torn

1 cup of fresh parsley, torn

2 cups of broccoli, trimmed

1 large green apple, chopped

1 cup of fresh spinach, torn

2 oz of water

Preparation:

Combine kale, parsley, and spinach in a colander and wash under cold running water. Drain and torn with hands. Set aside.

Wash the broccoli under cold running water and cut into small pieces. Set aside.

Wash the apple and cut in half. Remove the core and cut into bite-sized pieces. Set aside.

Now, combine kale, parsley, broccoli, apple, and spinach in a juicer. Process until well juiced and stir in the water.

Refrigerate for 10 minutes before serving.

Nutrition information per serving: Kcal: 223, Protein: 20.4g, Carbs: 62.1g, Fats: 3.5g

45.   Apple Strawberry Juice

Ingredients:

1 large red apple, cored

2 large strawberries, chopped

2 large grapefruits, peeled

1 small ginger knob, peeled

2 oz of coconut water

Preparation:

Wash the apple and cut in half. Remove the core and cut into bite-sized pieces. Set aside.

Wash the strawberries and cut into small pieces. Set aside.

Peel the grapefruits and divide into wedges. Set aside.

Peel the ginger knob and set aside.

Now, combine apple, strawberries, grapefruit, and ginger in a juicer. Process until well juiced and transfer to serving glasses. Stir in the coconut water and refrigerate for 10 minutes before serving.

Enjoy!

Nutrition information per serving: Kcal: 302, Protein: 4.8g, Carbs: 86.3g, Fats: 1.7g

46.　　Cucumber Swiss Chard Juice

Ingredients:

1 large cucumber, sliced

1 cup of Swiss chard, torn

2 cups of pumpkin, cubed

1 large green apple, cored

2 oz of water

¼ tsp of nutmeg, ground

Preparation:

Wash the cucumber and cut into thin slices. Set aside.

Wash the Swiss chard thoroughly under cold running water. Drain and torn with hands. Set aside.

Peel the pumpkin and cut in half. Scoop out the seeds using a spoon. Cut one large wedge and peel it. Cut into small cubes and fill the measuring cup. Reserve the rest for some other juice.

Wash the apple and cut in half. Remove the core and cut into bite-sized pieces. Set aside.

Now, combine pumpkin, apple, cucumber, and Swiss

chards in a juicer. Process until well juiced and stir in the water and nutmeg.

Refrigerate for 10 minutes before serving.

Nutrition information per serving: Kcal: 196, Protein: 5.8g, Carbs: 55.4g, Fats: 1.1g

47.   Bean Mint Juice

Ingredients:

1 cup of green beans, chopped

1 cup of fresh mint, torn

2 cups of celery, chopped

1 cup of beet greens, torn

1 large cucumber, sliced

2 oz of water

¼ tsp of salt

Preparation:

Wash the green beans and cut into bite-sized pieces. Soak in hot water for 10 minutes. Drain and set aside.

Wash the celery and cut into small pieces. Set aside.

Combine mint and beet greens in a colander. Wash under cold running water and torn with hands. Set aside.

Wash the cucumber and cut into thin slices. Set aside.

Now, combine green beans, mint, celery, beet greens, and cucumber in a juicer. Process until well juiced and transfer to a serving glass. Stir in the water and salt.

Refrigerate for 5 minutes before serving.

Nutritional information per serving: Kcal: 91, Protein: 6.1g, Carbs: 26.1g, Fats: 1g

48.   Lemon Kiwi Juice

Ingredients:

1 large lemon, peeled

1 large kiwi, peeled

1 cup of strawberries, chopped

2 large peaches, pitted

1 large green apple, cored

1 large orange, peeled

2 oz of water

Preparation:

Peel the lemon and kiwi. Cut lengthwise in half and set aside.

Wash the strawberries under cold running water. Remove the green parts and cut into bite-sized pieces. Set aside.

Wash the peaches and cut in half. Remove the pits and cut into small pieces. Set aside.

Wash the apple and cut half. Remove the core and cut into bite-sized pieces. Set aside.

Now, combine, lemon, kiwi, strawberries, peaches, and apple in a juicer and process until well juiced. Transfer to serving glasses and stir in the water. Add some ice and serve immediately.

Enjoy!

Nutrition information per serving: Kcal: 345, Protein: 7.8g, Carbs: 105g, Fats: 2.3g

49.   Raspberry Apricot Juice

Ingredients:

1 cup of raspberries

3 large apricots, pitted

1 cup of blackberries

1 large red apple, cored

3 large carrots, peeled

Preparation:

Combine raspberries and blackberries in a colander. Wash under cold running water and slightly drain. Set aside.

Wash the apricots and cut in half. Remove the pits and cut into bite-sized pieces. Set aside.

Wash the apple and cut in half. Remove the core and cut into small pieces.

Wash and peel the carrots. Cut into thin slices and set aside.

Now, combine blackberries, raspberries, apricots, apple, and carrots in a juicer. Process until well juiced and transfer to serving glasses. Stir in the water and refrigerate for 10

minutes before serving.

Enjoy!

Nutrition information per serving: Kcal: 301, Protein: 7.6g, Carbs: 97.4g, Fats: 2.9g

50.   Avocado Mint Juice

Ingredients:

1 cup of avocado, pitted

1 cup of fresh mint, chopped

1 cup of strawberries, chopped

1 large Granny Smith's apple, cored and chopped

1 large lemon, peeled

1 large cucumber, sliced

Preparation:

Peel the avocado and cut lengthwise in half. Remove the pit and cut into chunks and fill the measuring cup. Reserve the rest for later.

Wash the mint thoroughly and torn with hands. Set aside.

Wash the strawberries and cut into small pieces. Set aside.

Wash the apple and cut in half. Remove the core and cut into bite-sized pieces. Set aside.

Peel the lemon and cut lengthwise in half. Set aside.

Wash the cucumber and cut into thin slices. Set aside.

Now, combine avocado, mint, strawberries, lemon, and cucumber in a juicer and process until juiced. Transfer to serving glasses and stir in the water. Add some ice and serve immediately.

Nutrition information per serving: Kcal: 376, Protein: 8.1g, Carbs: 67.8g, Fats: 23.3g

51.　Cranberry Plum Juice

Ingredients:

1 cup of cranberries

4 whole plums, pitted

1 cup of pomegranate seeds

1 large red bell pepper, chopped

1 large green apple, cored

Preparation:

Wash the cranberries thoroughly and drain. Set aside.

Wash the plums and cut in half. Remove the pits and cut into bite-sized pieces. Set aside.

Cut the top of the pomegranate fruit using a sharp knife. Slice down to each of the white membranes inside of the fruit. Pop the seeds into a measuring cup and set aside.

Wash the bell pepper and cut lengthwise in half. Remove the seeds and cut into small pieces. Set aside.

Wash the apple and cut in half. Remove the core and cut into bite-sized pieces. Set aside.

Now, combine cranberries, plums, pomegranate, and

apple in a juicer. Process until well juiced and add some ice before serving.

Enjoy!

Nutrition information per serving: Kcal: 277, Protein: 6g, Carbs: 83g, Fats: 1.4g

52.   Blueberry Cucumber Juice

Ingredients:

1 cup of blueberries

1 large cucumber, sliced

1 cup of mango, chopped

1 large green apple, cored

2 oz of water

Preparation:

Place the blueberries in a colander and wash under cold running water. Drain and set aside.

Wash the cucumber and cut into thin slices. Set aside.

Wash the mango and cut into chunks. Fill the measuring cup and reserve the rest for some other juice. Set aside.

Wash the apple and remove the core. Cut into bite-sized pieces and set aside.

Now, combine blueberries, cucumber, mango, and apple in a juicer and process until juiced.

Transfer to serving glasses and stir in the water. Add some ice before serving and enjoy!

Nutrition information per serving: Kcal: 180, Protein: 5.9g, Carbs: 63.5g, Fats: 1.1g

53.   Celery Mint Juice

Ingredients:

1 cup of celery, chopped

1 cup of fresh mint, chopped

1 large lemon, peeled

1 cup of fresh spinach, chopped

2 oz of water

Preparation:

Wash the celery stalks and chop into small pieces. Fill the measuring cup and set aside. Peel the lemon and cut lengthwise in half. Set aside. Wash the spinach and mint in a colander. Chop and place in a medium bowl. Set aside. Now, combine celery, lemon, mint, and spinach in a juicer and process until juiced. Transfer to serving glasses and stir in the water. Refrigerate for 5 minutes before serving.

Nutrition information per serving: Kcal: 35, Protein: 3.1g, Carbs: 13.2g, Fats: 0.7g

MEALS

1.   Barley Porridge

Ingredients:

½ cup of barley, cooked

1 cup of almond milk

1 tbsp of honey

A handful of fresh dates, finely chopped

1 tbsp of fresh lemon juice

1 tbsp of almonds, finely chopped

Preparation:

Soak barley overnight. Drain and place in a deep pot. Add about two cups of water and bring it to a boil. Cook for 15 minutes over medium temperature. Remove from the heat, drain and cool for a while.

Transfer to a powerful food processor. Add fresh dates and pulse until well incorporated.

Place in a serving bowl, add almond milk, one tablespoon

of lemon juice, and top with finely chopped almonds. Stir in one tablespoon of honey and serve.

Nutrition information per serving: Kcal: 172, Protein: 15.5g, Carbs: 48.8g, Fats: 1.2g

2.   Greek Yogurt with Cranberries

Ingredients:

1 ½ cup of Greek yogurt

1 large banana

¼ cup of cranberries

1 tsp of vanilla sugar

1 tbsp of honey

Preparation:

Peel and roughly chop the banana. Mash well with a fork and transfer to a food processor. Add Greek yogurt, vanilla sugar, and honey. Pulse well to combine and pour into a bowl.

Stir in cranberries and serve.

Nutrition information per serving: Kcal: 199, Protein: 17g, Carbs: 31.2g, Fats: 8.6g

3.   Green Apple Overnight Oats with Raisins

Ingredients:

4 tbsp of rolled oats

1 tbsp of raisins

1 cup of skim milk

1 small green apple, peeled and chopped

1 tbsp of honey

Preparation:

In a medium-sized bowl, combine rolled oats with milk. Stir in honey and refrigerate overnight.

Stir in one tablespoon of raisins and top with chopped apple before serving.

You can add about ½ tsp of cinnamon, but this is optional.

Nutrition information per serving: Kcal: 322, Protein: 7.3g, Carbs: 60.6g, Fats: 8.1g

4.   Matcha Banana Pudding

Ingredients:

2 large bananas, peeled and chopped

1 ½ tsp of Matcha

1 cup of Greek yogurt (can be replaced with almond yogurt)

2 tbsp of honey

2 tbsp of freshly squeezed lemon juice

Preparation:

Combine the ingredients in a food processor and mix for 30 seconds.

Place the mixture in a bowl and refrigerate overnight.

Serve cold.

Nutrition information per serving: Kcal: 195, Protein: 3.6g, Carbs: 39.5g, Fats: 3.6g

5.   Warm Barley Cereal with Strawberries

Ingredients:

1 cup of quick-cooking barley

3 cups of skim milk

1 tbsp of ground flax meal

¼ tsp of salt

¼ cup of strawberry jam

4-5 fresh strawberries, sliced

1 tbsp of almonds, chopped

Preparation:

In a large saucepan, stir together quick-cooking barley, skim milk, one tablespoon of ground flax meal, and salt. Bring to a boil and reduce the heat to medium. Simmer for ten minutes. Remove from the heat and cool for a while.

Stir in strawberry jam and almonds. Top with fresh strawberries and serve.

Nutrition information per serving: Kcal: 122, Protein: 2.5g, Carbs: 26.7g, Fats: 1.8g

6.   Creamy Baked Zucchini with Thyme

Ingredients:

1 medium-sized zucchini, sliced into one inch thick slices

2 large tomatoes, sliced into one inch thick slices

1 large red bell pepper, sliced into one inch thick slices

5 tbsp of Greek yogurt

1 garlic clove, crushed

1 tsp of dried thyme

3 whole eggs

3 tbsp of whole milk

1 ½ tbsp of parmesan cheese, grated

½ tsp of salt

¼ tsp of pepper

3 tbsp of olive oil

Preparation:

Preheat the oven to 350 degrees.

Grease one (9x13-inch) casserole pan with olive oil and set

aside.

In a small bowl, stir together Greek yogurt, crushed garlic, and parmesan cheese.

In another bowl, whisk together eggs, milk, and dred thyme.

Now place zucchini in a casserole dish. Make another layer with tomatoes, and finish with red bell pepper. Spread Greek yogurt mixture over it and bake for 30 minutes.

Remove from the oven and gently spread the egg mixture using a kitchen brush.

Place in the oven for 3 more minutes and serve.

Nutrition information per serving: Kcal: 150, Protein: 7.9g, Carbs: 7.3g, Fats: 12.2g

7.   Warm Mussel Risotto with Rosemary

Ingredients:

1 cup of rice

7oz mussels

1 small onion, finely chopped

1 garlic clove, crushed

1 tbsp of dry rosemary, finely chopped

¼ cup of salted capers

1 tsp of chili pepper, ground

½ tsp of salt

3 tbsp of olive oil

4 salted anchovies

Preparation:

Place the rice in a deep pot. Add three cups of water and bring it to a boil. Cook for 15 minutes, stirring occasionally.

Heat up the olive oil over medium heat. Add finely chopped onion and garlic. Stir-fry until translucent. Now add the mussels, rosemary, chili pepper, and salt. Continue to cook for 7-10 minutes. Remove from the heat and combine with rice.

Add capers, top with anchovies, and mix well.

Serve!

Nutrition information per serving: Kcal: 187 Protein: 4g, Carbs: 39g, Fats: 17g

8. Cold Tomato Couscous

Ingredients:

5 oz of couscous

3 tbsp of tomato sauce

3 tbsp of lemon juice

1 small-sized onion, chopped

1 cup of vegetable stock

½ small-sized cucumber,sliced

½ small-sized carrot, sliced

¼ tsp of chili powder

¼ tsp of salt

¼ tsp of black pepper

3 tbsp of olive oil

½ cup of fresh parsley, chopped

Preparation:

First, pour the couscous into a large bowl. Boil the vegetable broth and slightly add it the couscous while stirring constantly. Leave it for about 10 minutes until couscous absorbs the liquid. Cover with a lid and set aside. Stir from time to time to speed up the soaking process and break the lumps with a spoon.

Meanwhile, preheat the olive oil in a frying pan, and add the tomato sauce. Add chopped onion and stir until translucent. Set aside and let it cool for few minutes.

Add the oily tomato sauce to the couscous and stir well. Now add lemon juice,chopped parsley, chili powder, salt, and pepper to the mixture and give it a final stir.

Serve with sliced cucumber, carrot, and parsley.

Nutrition information per serving: Kcal: 261, Protein: 8.2g, Carbs: 38.8g, Fats: 7.4g

9.   Lean Beef and Eggplant Stew

Ingredients:

7oz lean beef, chopped into bite sized pieces

1 eggplant, sliced

1 medium-sized onion, peeled and chopped

2 large, fresh tomatoes, roughly chopped

1 large potato, chopped

7.5 oz green beans

3.5 oz cabbage, shredded

1 medium-sized chili pepper

2 stalks of celery

3 tbsp of olive oil

1 tbsp of red wine vinegar

Salt to taste

1 tsp of sugar

½ tbsp of basil, dry

Preparation:

Chop the eggplants into bite-sized pieces and season with some salt. Allow it to stand for about 5 minutes and rinse well.

Meanwhile, heat up the olive oil over a medium heat. Add the onions and stir-fry for 2-3 minutes. Now add celery, basil, sugar, salt, vinegar, and tomatoes. Continue to cook for 2 more minutes.

Transfer to a deep pot and add other ingredients. Add about one cup of water and cook for about 20 minutes over high temperature.

Nutrition information per serving: Kcal: 198 Protein: 38g, Carbs: 27g, Fats: 19g

10. Creamy Yogurt Wraps with Ripe Tomatoes

Ingredients:

8oz chicken breast, boneless and skinless, cut into bite-sized pieces

½ medium-sized bell pepper, finely chopped

½ cup of red beans, cooked

3 large ripe tomatoes, roughly chopped

3 tbsp of extra-virgin olive oil

½ tsp of dry oregano

1 tsp of sugar

1 tsp of ground cumin

¼ cup of fresh parsley, finely chopped

½ cucumber, sliced

1 cup of thick yogurt

4 round tortillas (you can use pita breads instead)

Preparation:

Heat up the olive oil in a medium-sized skillet, over medium heat. Add chopped tomato and stir-fry for about five minutes, or until the liquid has evaporated. Now add oregano, cumin, and sugar. Mix well, cover, and set aside.

Meanwhile, heat up some more olive oil. Add chopped chicken and stir-fry for ten minutes, stirring constantly.

Sprinkle some water over each tortilla and warm them up in a microwave. If you're using pita breads, just warm them up.

Spread the tomato mixture over each tortilla and add sliced cucumber, chopped meat, bell pepper, and red beans. Top with yogurt and parsley. Serve!

Nutrition information per serving: Kcal: 270, Protein: 39g, Carbs: 31g, Fats: 13g

11.   Sweet Potato Patties with Fig Jam

Ingredients:

1lb sweet potato, peeled

8oz all-purpose flour plus 4oz more for dough

2oz wheat grits

1 egg yolk

2oz butter, melted

1 tsp of salt

Filling:

8oz unsweetened fig jam

4oz butter

1.5oz breadcrumbs

Other:

Powdered sugar

Preparation:

Gently peel the sweet potato and slice into one inch thick slices. Place in a deep pot and add enough water to cover. Bring it to a boil and cook until soften. This should take about five minutes because sweet potato takes less time to soften.

Remove from the heat and drain. Mash into a smooth puree. You can use a food processor for this to save yourself some time. Transfer to a bowl. Add 8oz flour, wheat grits, yolk, salt and butter. If you're using a food processor, the entire process will be much easier. If not, mash well with a fork and make a smooth dough-like mixture.

Roll the dough out until approximately 1-5 inches thick. Cut into 2-inches thick squares. Place one teaspoon of fig jam into each sqare, cover with another one, and tightly press the edges.

Place patties into a deep pot and add enough water to cover. Cook for 15 minutes over a medium heat. Remove from the heat and drain. Cool for a while.

Meanwhile, melt the butter in a large saucepan. Add breadcrumbs and briefly fry for 2-3 minutes.

Sprinkle breadcrumbs over patties and add some powdered sugar.

Serve.

Nutrition information per serving: Kcal: 182, Protein: 1.5g, Carbs: 27.5g, Fats: 8.4g

12.   Slow-Cooked Ginger Chicken

Ingredients:

2 pounds chicken thighs (skin and bones should be left on)

1 tablespoon chili powder

Fresh basil

Black pepper, freshly ground

Sea salt

16 ounces coconut water

1 tablespoon grated ginger, fresh

1 tablespoon coriander seeds

8 peeled and lightly smashed garlic cloves

Preparation:

Put the chicken thighs along with garlic in the slow cooker. Add rest of the spices, sprinkling them evenly over the chicken thighs. Pour the coconut water on the thighs and add the fresh basil. Cover the slow cooker and set the heat to low. You need to cook the thighs for around 3 to 4 hours before they are tender enough to eat. The liquid will also give off an enticing aroma when the ginger chili chicken is ready.

Nutrition information per serving: Kcal: 301 Protein: 33.2g, Carbs: 3.2g, Fats: 15.4g

13.   Southern Lamb Stew

Ingredients:

3lbs lamb cutlets

10 dried chilies

1 ½ tsp of salt

4 Japones chilies

1 ttbsp ground cumin

3 cups water

1 quartered large yellow onion

5 crushed garlic cloves

Preparation:

Take a sharp knife and slice each chili down the middle. Make sure you cut it into two neat halves so the seeds and the stems of the chilies can be removed easily. Take a small saucepan and toss the chilies into it. Put in all the spices along with the garlic and onion. Then, pour 3 cups of water into the saucepan. Turn the heat up to high and bring the mixture to a boil. Once boiled, let it cool for 10 minutes.

Take 2 cups of the mixture from the saucepan along with

garlic, onion and chilies and put in a blender. Puree the mixture till it turns completely smooth. Take the lamb cutlets and put it in the pot. Pour the mixture in the blender over the cutlets, set the heat to medium and let it cook for 1 hour. Stir the sauce properly and shred the cutlets before serving.

Nutrition information per serving: Kcal: 135 Protein: 15.62g, Carbs: 5g, Fats: 8.31g

14.   Wild Salmon Salad

Ingredients:

2 medium-sized cucumbers, sliced

A handful of Iceberg lettuce, torn

¼ cup of sweet corn

1 large tomato, roughly chopped

8oz smoked wild salmon, sliced

4 tbsp of freshly squeezed orange juice

Dressing:

1 ¼ cup of liquid yogurt, 2% fat

¼ cup of fat-free mayonnaise

1 tbsp of fresh mint, finely chopped

2 garlic cloves, crushed

1 tbsp of sesame seeds

Preparation:

Combine vegetables in a large bowl. Drizzle with orange juice and top with salmon slices. Set aside.

In another bowl, whisk together yogurt, mayonnaise, mint, crushed garlic, and sesame seeds.

Drizzle over salad and toss to combine. Serve cold.

Nutrition information per serving: Kcal: 521, Protein: 32.2g, Carbs: 63.5g, Fats: 24.3g

15.   Fresh Italian Parsley Pasta with Seafood

Ingredients:

1 pack of any pasta you like

1 pound of frozen seafood mix

4 tbsp of olive oil

2 garlic cloves, crushed

1 small onion, peeled and finely chopped

½ tsp of dry oregano

¼ tsp of salt

¼ cup of white wine

Preparation:

Use the package instructions to prepare pasta. Rinse well and drain. Set aside.

Heat up the olive oil over a medium temperature. Add the onion and garlic and stir-fry for several minutes, or until translucent. Now add seafood mix, oregano, wine and salt. Reduce the heat to low and cook until the seafood mix have softened. You might want to check the octopus as it takes the most time to soften. Turn off the heat, add pasta and cover. Let it stand for 10 minutes before serving.

Nutritional values: Kcal: 315 Protein: 20g, Carbs: 42g, Fats: 8g

16. Pide Bread with Stewed Veggies

Ingredients:

7oz lean ground beef

½ small green pepper, finely chopped

½ small red bell pepper, finely chopped

1 large tomato, peeled and chopped

1 small onion, finely chopped

½ cup of grated gouda cheese

4 tbsp of extra virgin olive oil

1 tsp of cayenne pepper, ground

1 tsp of chili pepper, ground

½ tsp of salt

1 pide bread

Preparation:

Preheat the oven to 350 degrees.

Heat up two tablespoons of olive oil over medium temperature. Stir-fry the onion for 2 minutes and add finely chopped green and red pepper. Continue to cook for one more minute and add meat. Cook for ten minutes and remove from the heat.

Spread the meat mixture over the pide bread, add chopped tomato, grated gouda cheese, cayenne pepper, chili pepper, and salt. Top with two tablespoons of olive oil and bake for 5 minutes.

Serve warm.

Nutrition information per serving: Kcal: 369, Protein: 30g, Carbs: 58g, Fats: 24g

17.   Ground Beef Cannelloni

Ingredients:

1 pack of cannelloni (8.8oz)

2 medium-sized red onions, finely chopped

1 pound of lean ground beef

½ tsp of salt

¼ tsp of freshly ground black pepper

3 tbsp of vegetable oil

Preparation:

Heat up the vegetable oil over a medium temperature. Stir-fry the onions for 3 minutes and add ground beef. Stir well and continue to cook for another ten minutes. Use the mixture to fill cannelloni.

Place in the oven for 20 minutes, or until golden brown.

Nutritional information per serving: Kcal: 417, Protein: 47g, Carbs: 43.5g, Fats: 24g

18.   Lean Spring Stew

Ingredients:

1 pound diced fire roasted tomatoes

4 boneless & skinless chicken thighs

1 tablespoon dried basil

8 ounces chicken stock

Salt & pepper

4 ounces tomato paste

3 chopped celery stalks

3 chopped carrots

2 chili peppers, finely chopped

2 tablespoons olive oil

1 finely chopped onion

2 garlic cloves, crushed

½ container mushrooms

Sour cream

Preparation:

Heat up the olive oil over a medium-high temperature. Add the celery, onions and carrots and stir-fry for 5 to 10 minutes. Transfer to a deep pot and add tomato paste, basil, garlic, mushrooms and seasoning. Keep stirring the vegetables till they are completely covered by tomato sauce. At the same time, cut the chicken into small cubes to make it easier to eat.

Put the chicken in a deep pot, pour the chicken stock over it and throw in the tomatoes. Stir the chicken in to ensure the ingredients and vegetables are properly mixed with it. Turn the heat to low and cook for about an hour. The vegetables and chicken should be cooked through before you turn the heat off. Top with sour cream and serve!

Nutrition information per serving: Kcal: 291Protein:27g, Carbs: 37g, Fats: 3g

19.   Stewed Beef with Olives

Ingredients:

2 pounds of ground beef

1 onion, peeled and chopped

2 chili peppers, finely chopped and seeds removed

3 garlic cloves, crushed

2 tsp of cumin, ground

2 tbsp of apple cider vinegar

28 oz of fire-roasted tomatoes

Salt to taste

½ tsp of cinnamon, ground

Oil for frying

For serving:

¼ cup of green olives

1 tbsp of raisins

1 tbsp of toasted almonds

Preparation:

Heat up about three tablespoons of oil over a medium-high temperature. Add garlic, onion and chili peppers. Stir-fry for about five minutes and add cumin and cinnamon. Mix well and cook for another minute.

Season the meat with some salt and place in a frying skillet. Stir-fry for several minutes and then add other ingredients. Bring it to a boil and reduce the heat. Simmer for about 10 minutes.

Top with green olives, toasted almonds and raisins.

Nutrition information per serving: Kcal: 521 Protein: 38g, Carbs: 29.5g, Fats: 15g

20.   Red Orange Salad

Ingredients:

Fresh lettuce leaves, rinsed

1 small cucumber sliced

½ red bell pepper, sliced

1 cup of frozen seafood mix

1 onion, peeled and finely chopped

3 garlic cloves, crushed

¼ cup of fresh orange juice

5 tbsp of extra virgin olive oil

Salt to taste

Preparation:

Heat up 3 tbsp of extra virgin olive oil over medium-high temperature. Add chopped onion and crushed garlic. Stir fry for about 5 minutes. Reduce the heat to minimum and add 1 cup of frozen seafood mix. Cover and cook for about 15 minutes, until soft. Remove from the heat and allow it to cool for a while.

Meanwhile, combine the vegetables in a bowl. Add the

remaining 2 tbsp of olive oil, fresh orange juice and little salt. Toss well to combine.

Top with seafood mix and serve immediately.

Nutrition information per serving: Kcal: 286, Protein: 34.5g, Carbs: 28g, Fats: 26g

21.   Lean Beef Rolls

Ingredients:

1 cup of rice

1 pound of ground beef

¼ cup of finely chopped tomato

¼ cup of finely chopped red bell pepper

1 tbsp of tomato paste

1 tbsp of chili pepper, ground

1 chili pepper, finely diced

½ tsp of salt

¼ tsp of pepper

1 tbsp of fresh lime juice

1 bunch of collard greens

1 cup of cream for serving

1 tbsp of butter

Preparation:

Briefly boil the collard greens (2 minutes will be enough).

Remove from the heat and drain. Set aside.

Meanwhile, in a large bowl combine the ingredients and mix well. Use one tbsp of this mixture for each roll. Melt the butter in a deep pot and place the rolls. Add about ¼ cup of water, cover the pot and cook for about 30 minutes over medium temperature.

Serve with cream, cheese or yogurt.

Nutrition information per serving: Kcal: 151 Protein: 49g, Carbs: 19.1g, Fats: 9g

22.　　Cliantro Bean Salad

Ingredients:

1 cup of cooked beans

½ cup of sweet corn

3 spring onions, chopped

¼ small chili pepper, finely chopped

¼ tsp of cliantro

½ tsp of red wine vinegar

1 tsp of fresh lemon juice

3 tbsp of extra-virgin olive oil

A pinch of salt

Preparation:

In a small bowl, combine the olive oil with red wine vinegar, fresh lemon juice, cliantro, and a pinch of salt. Mix well and use to season the other ingredients.

Serve!

Nutrition information per serving: Kcal: 151 Protein: 49g, Carbs: 19.1g, Fats: 9g

23.   Chili Salad with Peppers

Ingredients:

1 cup of white beans

1 red bell pepper, chopped

1 tsp of ground chili pepper

1 tsp of parsley, finely chopped

1 tbsp of olive oil

1 tsp of lemon juice

½ tsp of sea salt

Preparation:

Wash and peel the pepper. Chop into bite size pieces. Mix with beans in a large bowl and top with olive oil, lemon juice and salt. Serve cold.

Nutrition information per serving: Kcal: 95 Protein: 5.9g, Carbs: 11.8g, Fats: 5g

24. Leafy Chicken Breast Salad

Ingredients:

1 piece of chicken breast, 0.5 inch thick, boneless and skinless

1 cup of finely chopped lettuce

Several spinach leaves

½ cup of beans, pre-cooked

1 tbsp of fresh lime juice

1 tsp of ground chili

1 tbsp of vegetable oil

Pinch of salt

Preparation:

Preheat a non-stick grill pan over a medium-high temperature. Wash and pat dry the meat using a kitchen paper. Grill for about 4-5 minutes on each side. You can use some water if necessary. Several tablespoons at a time will be enough to make the process easier. Remove from the heat and cut into several pieces.

Combine the meat with other ingredients, toss with

vegetable oil, fresh lime juice, and a pinch of salt. Serve.

Nutrition information per serving: Kcal: 189 Protein: 31g, Carbs: 24g, Fats: 12g

25.   Northern Bean Soup

Ingredients:

1 pound of dried great northern beans

¾ cup of onions, peeled and finely chopped

½ tbsp of vegetable oil

½ tbsp of cumin, ground

½ tbps of oregano, dry

Salt and pepper to taste

4 cups of chicken broth

1 garlic clove, crushed

1 pound of chicken breast, boneless and skinless

4 ounce can of green chillies, chopped

Preparation:

Place the beans in a deep pot. Add enough water to cover and bring it to a boil. Cook for several minutes and remove from the heat. Cover and let it stand for several hours until soften. Drain and rinse well.

Heat up some oil in a frying skillet. Add the onion and stir-fry for about one minute. Now add the beans, crushed garlic and chicken broth. Reduce the heat and cook for about two hours.

Preheat the oven to 350 degrees. Place the ingredients in a baking dish and coat well. Cover and cook for about an hour. Serve warm.

Nutrition information per serving: Kcal: 111 Protein: 8.1g, Carbs: 25.4g, Fats: 8g

26.   Cliantro Lentil Stew with Carrots

Ingredients:

10oz lentils

1.5 tbsp of butter

1 medium-sized carrot, peeled and sliced

1 small potato, peeled and chopped

1 bay leaf

¼ cup of parsley, finely chopped

½ tbsp of fresh cliantro

Salt to taste

Preparation:

Melt the butter in a medium-sized skillet. Add sliced carrot, chopped potato and parsley. Mix well and stir-fry for about five minutes.

Now add the lentils, 1 bay leaf, some salt and cliantro. Add about 4 cups of water and bring it to a boil. Reduce the heat, cover and cook until the lentils soften.

Sprinkle with some parsley before serving.

Nutrition information per serving: Kcal: 313 Protein: 36g, Carbs: 42.1g, Fats: 28g

27.   Lean Spring Veggie Risotto

Ingredients:

1 cup of rice

½ cup of green beans, pre-cooked

2 medium-sized red bell peppers, finely chopped

1 medium-sized zucchini, sliced

1 pice of chicken breast, boneless and skinless

3 tbsp of extra virgin olive oil

½ tsp of salt

Preparation:

Place the rice in a deep pot. Add 2 cups of water and bring it to a boil. Reduce the heat and cook until the water evaporates. Stir occasionally.

Stir in the olive oil, salt, sliced zucchini, green beans, and peppers. Add one cup of water and continue to cook for another 10 minutes.

Meanwhile, heat up a non-stick frying pan. Place the chicken breast and cover. Cook for 15 minutes, or until the meat has softened. Serve with rice.

Nutrition information per serving: Kcal: 220 Protein: 8g, Carbs: 45g, Fats: 3g

28. Sweet Pumpkin Soup

Ingredients:

21oz sweet pumpkin meat, chopped

2 medium-sized onions, peeled and finely chopped

1 garlic clove

1 red pepper, finely chopped

1 tbsp of fresh tomato sauce

½ tbsp of chili powder

2 bay leaves

2 cups of red wine

1 cup of water

1 tsp of thyme, dry

Salt and pepper to taste

Oil for frying

Preparation:

Heat up some oil in a frying skillet and add the chopped onions. Stir-fry for two minutes and add finely chopped red pepper, tomato sauce, and chili powder. Continue to fry until the peper has softened. Add the remaining ingredients and bring it to a boil. Reduce the heat to minimum and cook for about an hour.

Remove from the heat and serve.

Nutrition information per serving: Kcal: 130 Protein: 24g, Carbs: 29g, Fats: 11g

29.   Almond Rice with Beans

Ingredients:

3 tbsp of olive oil

2 tbsp of vegetable oil

1 small onion, peeled and chopped

3 garlic cloves, crushed

28oz beans, pre-cooked

1 tsp of dry marjoram

1 small chili pepper, finely chopped

3 tbsp of Worcestershire sauce

1.7oz toasted almonds, chopped

A handful of pumpkin seeds for serving

1 cup of cooked rice, for serving

Preparation:

Combine the olive oil with vegetable oil and heat up over a medium-high temperature. Add chopped onion and garlic cloves. Stir-fry for 2-3 minutes and other ingredients. Pour about ¼ cup of water and cook for about 10 minutes, or until all the water has evaporated.

Remove from the heat and chill for a while. Serve with rice and top with pumpkin seeds.

Nutrition information per serving: Kcal: 113 Protein: 17g, Carbs: 35g, Fats: 16g

30. Vegetarian Pea Stew

Ingredients:

21oz peas, pre-cooked

1 medium-sized tomato, roughly chopped

1 medium-sized onion, peeled and sliced

2 large carrots, peeled and sliced

2 small potatoes, peeled and chopped

1 celery stalk

A handful of parsley, finely chopped

2 garlic cloves, crushed

2 bay leaves

4 tbsp of fresh tomato sauce

Olive oil

Preparation:

Preheat some olive oil over a medium-high temperature. Add the chopped onion and garlic. Stir-fry for several minutes and add the sliced carrot, fresh tomato paste and finely chopped celery. Cook for about ten minutes, stirring constantly. Reduce the heat to minimum and add other ingredients. Pour in about 4 cups of water and cover. Cook for about 45 minutes.

Serve warm.

Nutrition information per serving: Kcal: 186 Protein: 22g, Carbs: 38g, Fats: 23g

31.   Spicy Roasted Chicken Legs

Ingredients:

1lb chicken legs

1 cup of vegetable oil

1 tsp Cayenne pepper

1 tsp salt

1 tbsp dried rosemary, crushed

1 tbsp peppercorns

1 tsp brown sugar

Preparation:

Combine the spices with vegetable oil. Wash and pat dry chicken legs and soak them in this mixture. Refrigerate for about an hour.

Preheat the oven to 300 degrees.

Use some of the marinade to grease the baking sheet. Place the chicken legs, skin side up and cover with foil.

Roast for about an hour and remove the foil. Return to the oven and roast for another 15 minutes.

Nutrition information per serving: Kcal: 350 Protein: 51g, Carbs: 0g, Fats: 15g

32.   Orange Arugula Salad with Smoked Turkey

Ingredients:

3.5 oz arugula, torn

3.5 oz lamb's lettuce, torn

3.5 oz lettuce, torn

8 oz smoked turkey breast, chopped into bite-sized pieces

2 large oranges, peeled and sliced

For dressing:

¼ cup of Greek yogurt

3 tbsp of lemon juice

1 tsp of apple cider vinegar

¼ cup of olive oil

Preparation:

Combine vegetables in a large bowl. Add turkey breast and toss well. Now add sliced oranges and set aside.

Place Greek yogurt in a small bowl. Add lemon juice, apple cider, and olive oil. Whisk together until fully combined.

Drizzle over salad and serve.

Nutrition information per serving: Kcal: 271, Protein: 25.3g, Carbs: 21.8g, Fats: 7.5g

33.   Avocado Detox Smoothie

Ingredients:

½ avocado, peeled and roughly chopped

1 banana, peeled and chopped

Handful of baby spinach, torn

1 tbsp of honey

1 tsp of turmeric, ground

1 tbsp of flaxseed, ground

1 tbsp of goji berries

Preparation:

Place the ingredients in a blender and mix well for 20 seconds.

Serve cold.

Nutrition information per serving: Kcal: 298, Protein: 4.2g, Carbs: 35.6g, Fats: 0.9g

34. Sweet Melon Salad with Hazelnuts

Ingredients:

2oz toasted hazelnuts, chopped

1lb melon, cut into bite-sized pieces

3.5 oz fresh arugula, torn

5 oz fresh raspberries

Dressing:

3.5 oz fresh raspberries

3 tbsp of fresh lime juice

1 tbsp of vanilla sugar

3 tbsp of hazelnut oil

Preparation:

Combine melon, arugula, raspberries, and hazelnuts in a large bowl.

Place all dressing ingredients in a food processor. Pulse to combine and drizzle over salad.

Serve cold.

Nutrition information per serving: Kcal: 87, Protein: 0.8g, Carb 15.3g, Fats: 0.4g

35.   Marinated Turkey Breast

Ingredients:

1lb turkey breast, boneless and skinless

1 tbsp of olive oil

4 garlic cloves

2 tbsp of apple cider vinegar

5 tbsp of fresh parsley, finely chopped

1 tsp of oregano

½ tsp of salt

Preparation:

Wash and pat dry the meat. Set aside.

Combine all other ingredients in a large bowl. Place the meat in it and marinate for about an hour.

Preheat the grill pan and grill the meat for about ten minutes on each side. A good idea is to add some of the marinade while grilling – about one tablespoon will be enough.

Serve immediately.

Nutrition information per serving: Kcal: 131, Protein: 21.4g, Carb 3.7g, Fats: 3.5g

36. Oven Roasted Beans

Ingredients:

24oz beans, pre-cooked

1 large onion, peeled and finely chopped

2 spring onions, finely chopped

3 cloves of garlic, crushed

2 carrots, peeled and sliced

2 tbsp of ground chili

1 tbsp of ground turmeric

Preparation:

Preheat the oven to 350 degrees.

Combine the ingredients in a casserole dish. Add about three cups of water and mix well. Bake for 30 minutes.

Nutrition information per serving: Kcal: 180 Protein: 24g, Carbs: 32g, Fats: 21g

37.   Sweet Corn Quinoa with Lime Juice

Ingredients:

2 tbsp of olive oil

2 cloves of garlic, crushed

1 jalapeño chili pepper, finely chopped

1 cup of quinoa

1 cup of green beans, pre-cooked

1 medium-sized tomato, finely chopped

1 cup of sweet corn

1 tsp of cayenne pepper

1 avocado, peeled and cored

1 lime, juiced

A hanful of fresh coriander

Salt and pepper to taste

Preparation:

Preheat the olive oil over a medium temperature. Add finely chopped jalapeño chili pepper and garlic. Stir-fry for about one minute.

Now add quinoa, green beans, finely chopped tomato, corn, and chili powder. Reduce the heat and cover. Cook for about 20 minutes.

Meanwhile, clean the avocado and chop into bite-sized pieces. Combine with lime juice and fresh coriander. Add to the mixture and serve.

Nutrition information per serving: Kcal: 374 Protein: 31g, Carbs: 64g, Fats: 28g

38.   Citrus Spring Salad

Ingredients:

1 small onion, peeled and finely chopped

2 medium-sized tomatoes, chopped

1 cup of fresh cliantro, finely chopped

2 cups of tuna, drained

1 medium-sized lime, juiced

¼ tsp of sea salt

1/8 tsp of freshly ground black pepper

Preparation:

Combine tomatoes, cheese, onions, and cliantro in a large bowl. Stir in the lime juice and toss to combine.

Flake tuna into small pieces and season with salt and pepper. Place in a bowl.

Gently toss to evenly distribute the ingredients and serve.

Nutrition information per serving: Kcal: 165, Protein: 2.1g, Carb 17.5g, Fats: 11.2g

ADDITIONAL TITLES FROM THIS AUTHOR

70 Effective Meal Recipes to Prevent and Solve Being Overweight: Burn Fat Fast by Using Proper Dieting and Smart Nutrition

By Joe Correa CSN

48 Acne Solving Meal Recipes: The Fast and Natural Path to Fixing Your Acne Problems in Less Than 10 Days!

By Joe Correa CSN

41 Alzheimer's Preventing Meal Recipes: Reduce or Eliminate Your Alzheimer's Condition in 30 Days or Less!

By Joe Correa CSN

70 Effective Breast Cancer Meal Recipes: Prevent and Fight Breast Cancer with Smart Nutrition and Powerful Foods

By Joe Correa CSN